Cristine Coelho Cazeiro
Daniela Copetti

People's knowledge of first aid

Cristine Coelho Cazeiro
Daniela Copetti

People's knowledge of first aid

Brazilian scientific production

ScienciaScripts

Imprint

Cover image: www.ingimage.com

This book is a translation from the original published under ISBN 978-620-2-04176-8.

Publisher:
Sciencia Scripts
is a trademark of
Dodo Books Indian Ocean Ltd. and OmniScriptum S.R.L publishing group

120 High Road, East Finchley, London, N2 9ED, United Kingdom
Str. Armeneasca 28/1, office 1, Chisinau MD-2012, Republic of Moldova, Europe
Managing Directors: Ieva Konstantinova, Victoria Ursu
info@omniscriptum.com

Printed at: see last page
ISBN: 978-620-8-50432-8

"Your work will take up a large part of your life and the only way to be satisfied is to do what you believe is great work."

Steve Jobs

SUMMARY

This is a descriptive study with a qualitative approach based on a systematic review of the literature, the aim of which was to find out about Brazilian scientific production on laypeople's knowledge of first aid. Data was collected in February and March 2015 from the following online databases: Latin American and Caribbean Health Sciences (LILACS), *Scientific Electronic Library Online* (SciELO), Nursing Database (BDENF) and *Medical Literature Analysis and Retrieval System Online* (MEDLINE). After a thorough reading of the articles, the data analyzed was categorized into three categories: the lay public's knowledge of first aid; means of disseminating information; and lines of action for health education. It emerged that studies on lay people's knowledge of first aid are scarce, and that the published studies involved only a few specific groups and did not provide a general overview. The selected studies showed that the subjects had incorrect or incomplete information about first aid. Strategies for health education included adapting the means of communication, locations and terms to the target audience in order to improve understanding and retention of knowledge, as well as starting information activities from childhood at school. There is a need for further studies focusing on laypeople's knowledge of first aid involving other audiences.

Keywords: knowledge; first aid; emergencies; nursing

SUMMARY

Chapter 1	4
Chapter 2	6
Chapter 3	13
Chapter 4	16
Chapter 5	34

1. INTRODUCED

The topic of First Aid or Pre-hospital Care is a frequent one in national and international literature. However, most of the time, it is related to the knowledge, skills or training of health professionals or students, and is rarely addressed to other audiences.

The lay public, often ignored by scholars in the field, is the one who will often witness urgent and emergency situations and provide first aid, either through the instinctive impulse to help others or because of the need due to the delay in the arrival of the rescue service due to bureaucratic issues and travel.

The need for training in first aid is also seen as necessary only for health professionals, mainly in urgent and emergency services. However, recent studies have highlighted the importance of training other audiences of different age groups through health education, with the aim of reducing injuries and maintaining life in emergency situations which are always, or almost always, unpredictable.

The effectiveness of first aid measures in emergency situations, regardless of the location of the incident and who is at the scene, can be decisive for the survival of victims and the reduction of sequelae. Therefore, it is essential to train the population in this area.

The main primers and manuals on first aid refer to the need for specific training for the lay public, including the American Heart Association's (AHA) Guidelines for Prehospital Care (APH) Manual, which has specific instructions for the lay first aider in each of its chapters, due to the relevance of instruction for this public.

There is no doubt that the subject is indeed relevant, but superficially, it can be seen that there are few bibliographic productions with this approach. In view of this, a more in-depth and systematic search is needed to find out what bibliographic production exists about the lay public's knowledge of first aid, thus characterizing the aim of this study.

Before carrying out any fieldwork, it is necessary and fundamental to obtain a complete overview of what has already been produced in the area, both to acquire a better scientific foundation and to confirm that fieldwork would really be contributing. With this in mind, the aim of this study was to identify the bibliographic production in Brazil on laypeople's knowledge of first aid.

2. THEORETICAL FRAMEWORK

2.1 EMERGENCIES AND FIRST AID

Emergency situations are defined by the World Health Organization (WHO) as risk situations with immediate consequences for life, which can be caused by natural phenomena, human acts, diseases or a combination of causes[1].

These episodes consist of immediate care that must be given quickly to a person. First aid performed objectively and effectively, with agility, dexterity and safety on victims of accidents or sudden illness, whose physical condition is life-threatening, requires the application of measures and procedures until qualified assistance arrives[3].

Knowledge and practice of first aid are essential for the patient to survive longer, thus maintaining vital functions, preventing their condition from worsening and reducing possible physical sequelae. Any previously trained individual will be able to identify the seriousness of the situation at an early stage, call the emergency team and carry out basic rescue maneuvers that can be decisive for the victim's survival.

The fact is that most of these situations occur in environments such as public roads, homes, schools and workplaces, where trained professionals and life support are not available, leaving whoever is at the scene to provide the first aid[4].

According to article 135 of the Brazilian Penal Code, failing to provide assistance, when it is possible to do so without personal risk, to a disabled or injured person who is helpless or in grave and imminent danger; or failing to call for help from the public authority is a crime[5].

Assistance is often provided inappropriately, through the impulse of solidarity by lay people, who, due to the emotional impact of the situation, often become victims themselves, or act hastily, which can worsen the victim's situation instead of helping them[2,6].

In-depth theoretical knowledge is not necessary for a person from the community, who is not a health professional, to be useful and effective at the time of an emergency. The action of a layperson who is able to quickly recognize a situation of Cardiorespiratory Arrest (CRA), for example, and immediately call for specialized help while performs chest compression maneuvers, prevents myocardial and cerebral deterioration, greatly increasing the victim's chance of survival without sequelae[7].

There is evidence of a reduction in mortality in victims of CPR who immediately received CPR maneuvers by volunteers and had their heart and brain functions preserved[7].

According to the American Heart Association, if CPR is performed in the first minute, the chances of success are up to 98%. From the fifth minute onwards, the chances of success drop to 25% and, if CPR is performed after ten minutes, the chance of the victim surviving drops to 1%[1].

Studies have shown that immediate CPR after collapse due to ventricular fibrillation can double or even triple the chances of survival. In contrast, the chances of survival decrease by 7-10% for every minute that CPR is delayed. (Clinical awareness) The proportion of this data contributes to the fact that cardiopulmonary arrest (CPR) is the leading cause of death in several countries, which reveals the importance of CPR in public health[9,10].

2.2 LIFE AND LIMB THREATENING SITUATIONS

Since the 1960s, cardiovascular diseases have been the leading cause of death in Brazil. Among them, ischemic heart disease is responsible for 80% of cardiac arrest episodes, most of which occur in out-of-hospital settings, where often the only immediate support is the action of those on the scene[10,11].

In addition to physiological causes (illnesses, sudden illness), external causes of mortality have been gaining prominence in Brazil. These are the second leading cause of death in the country, and the 5-39 age group is the main risk group[12].

According to the International Classification of Diseases (ICD), external causes include homicide, suicide, traffic accidents, poisoning, accidents at work, burns, falls, drowning, among others, which are popularly known as accidental causes[13].

Among them, traumatic injuries are one of the main causes of death and disability, occurring in all regions of the country, affecting individuals in all age groups and social classes, being responsible for around 60 million victims and three million deaths annually worldwide.These data correspond to one in six hospital admissions.In Brazil, mortality from trauma occupies the third position among the causes of death[2,6].

In Brazil alone, according to data from the Ministry of Health, 90,000 people die every year.

individuals due to trauma, most of them due to automobile accidents, and it is believed that many others will suffer permanent disability[14].

According to the World Health Organization (WHO), trauma is an international challenge for public health systems, and it is estimated that in 2020 traffic accidents will be the second leading external cause of mortality in the world[15].

Care for trauma victims, like other emergency situations, should begin as early as possible, with the best integration between care provided at the scene, care during transportation and definitive treatment[15].

It can be said that the success of all the other phases of treatment and rehabilitation, their future, their integrity as an individual, the presence or absence of sequelae and their post-accident quality of life depend on the first approach to the victim[3].

Despite its importance, the teaching of first aid is still not widespread among the general population, and learning is generally restricted to health professionals. It is essential that access to this knowledge is democratized and disseminated to society, allowing them to be able to act in emergency situations whenever necessary, since most of the time they are unpredictable and unexpected[4,16].

2.3 TRAINING THE COMMUNITY IN GENERAL IN FIRST AID

Training in Basic Life Support (BLS), due to its relevance to the rapid treatment of victims in emergency situations, is now a political strategy in the health care of the population. It includes interventions that can be carried out quickly by trained non-health professionals, which includes requesting

Advanced Life Support, as well as maneuvers to maintain airways and blood circulation[17].

The basic principles of first aid are: recognizing life-threatening situations, applying artificial respiration and circulation when necessary, controlling bleeding, minimizing the risk of other injuries or complications, avoiding infections, providing medical assistance and transport and making the victim as comfortable as possible[18].

Although several authors consider that basic life support maneuvers should be known not only by health professionals, but also by laypeople, this is still not a reality, which ends up causing many victims to suffer consequences that could have been avoided[18,19].

The ideal, according to Fioruc et al. (2008), is for all citizens to feel empowered to assess and conduct themselves in an emergency situation, having specific information on what to do in the event of an accident, which involves simple attitudes related to practicing first aid and also to the problems that can occur in order to prevent them[20].

In many situations, this lack of knowledge leads to numerous problems, such as panic at the sight of the injured person, incorrect handling of the victim and excessive and sometimes unnecessary requests for specialized emergency help[21].

Lay people, in their eagerness to help and also due to a lack of specific knowledge, when trying to help the victim, can contribute to worsening the situation, including irreversible damage. They often use common sense knowledge, to the detriment of what would be appropriate for certain situations[11].

In view of this, it is essential to educate and train the population in first aid, enabling them to act appropriately and avoid wasting time or being paralyzed by the emotions that an emergency situation triggers[7].

The need for educational interventions to this end should be emphasized more, as it is extremely necessary in our environment, where there are few or no first aid training programs for the lay community[22].

First aid techniques are indispensable, often making the difference between death and the continuation of life, and this is only possible when there are trained people capable of handling the situation calmly and confidently until the specialized service arrives[17].

In addition, it is essential that places such as schools, clubs, companies and other institutions maintain procedures in their day-to-day activities that make it easier to provide first aid, such as having information on how to behave in the event of an accident, spreading the word about who to look for and where to go, as well as being equipped with basic first aid materials[23].

3. METHODOLOGY

This research is characterized by a descriptive qualitative study, of the Systematic Literature Review type. This method consists of a form of research that uses bibliographic production on a given topic as its data source. This type of investigation provides a summary of the evidence related to a specific subject, through the application of rigorous and systematized methods of searching, critical appraisal and synthesis of the selected information.

A systematic review makes it possible to integrate information from a set of independently conducted studies that may present conflicting and/or coinciding results, as well as to identify topics that need more evidence, helping to guide future research[24].

Data was collected from the following online databases: Latin American and Caribbean Health Sciences (LILACS); *Sc/en////c Electronic Library Online* (SciELO); Nursing Database (BDENF) and *Medical Literature Analysis and Retrieval System Online* (MEDLINE) during the months of February and March 2015 using the following descriptors: First Aid, Emergencies and Knowledge.

The inclusion criteria used were: the study was available online for free on Integra; it was a scientific article, experience report or literature review published in a scientific journal; it dealt with the general public's knowledge of first aid and it was carried out in Brazil and had a Portuguese language version.

The exclusion criteria were: it was not an article (monograph, book, etc.); it was not available in Integra online; it did not deal with first aid knowledge or involve professionals or students from areas such as medicine, nursing, firefighters, professionals who theoretically receive specific training during their professional training; it was carried out abroad or did not contain a Portuguese language version, since at the moment, the interest is to identify the knowledge of the Brazilian lay public, which can differ greatly from that of foreigners. No time cut-off point was used.

The first stage of the search consisted of selecting the studies by title and abstract in each of the databases. Afterwards, a thorough reading of each study was carried out in order to identify the main results of each one and then formulate analytical categories, following the precepts of Minayo (2008)25.

3.1. ETHICAL ASPECTS

As this is a bibliographical search, this research did not require approval of the Ethics Committee. However, the principles of copyright were ensured by properly identifying the works and authors referenced.

4. RESULTS AND DISCUSSION

The table below summarizes the results of the search carried out in each of the databases consulted and the number of studies included and excluded with the appropriate justifications.

TABLE 1. Results of the bibliographic search, descriptors: First Aid; Emergencies; Knowledge

Database	No. of studies found	No. of people included	No. of excluded and justification
LILACS	16	4	9 because it deals with the knowledge of health professionals or students; 1 because it is a thesis; 1 for not having the full text available; 1 for not having text available in Portuguese.

SciELO	15	5	5 for not dealing with knowledge of first aid; 3 because it deals with the knowledge of health professionals or students; 2 for not having text available in Portuguese.
BDENF	5	1	2 for dealing with knowledge of health professionals or students; 2 because they were repeated studies, already found in other databases
MEDLINE	3	0	2 for not having the full text available; 1 for not having text available in Portuguese.

In total, 10 articles were analyzed. As expected, most of the studies referred to the knowledge of nursing or medical professionals or students, areas that deal directly with emergency situations in their work activities, with only a few studies involving other audiences.

Below is a brief summary of the studies included and the public involved:

TABLE 2: Included studies, main author, subjects, type and place of study

Main author	Audience/population	State/city	Type of study
Tomazin CC	Livestock farmers	Sumare-SP	Quantitative, cross-sectional
Fioruv BE	Teachers and staff from four public schools	Botucatu- SP	Quantitative, cross-sectional
Silva PO	40 teaching students medium	Cabo Frio- RJ	Qualitative descriptive
Goncalves AC	211 patients treated in the rehabilitation section of a burns service	Ribeirao Preto-SP	Qualitative descriptive
Ventorini JAO	10 Community Agents Health	A municipality in the northern region of Rio Grande do Sul	Qualitative descriptive
Pergola AM	385 lay people over the age of 18	A town in the interior of Sao Paulo	Quantitative cross-sectional
Mori S	First aid educational website	Sao Paulo- SP	Evaluation study
Veronese AM	A group of residents of a neighborhood	Porto Alegre-RS	Experience report

Andraus LMS	126 children aged 8 to 11	Goiania-GO	Experience report
Leitao FBP	47 health professionals and 59 members of the lay community (school teachers, hospital staff, engineers and scouts).	Sao Paulo-SP	Experience report

After a thorough reading of the articles found, the data analyzed was categorized into three categories, which are explored below:

4.1. THE LAY PUBLIC'S KNOWLEDGE OF FIRST AID

A lay rescuer is a person who has no professional training in the health field, but who can intervene in an emergency situation, helping to increase the survival and reduce the consequences of an accident victim or a life-threatening clinical situation[26].

Despite the existing evidence that the lay public is an important group in terms of first aid training, given that most accidents occur on public roads or in the home environment, with the public, family members or the victims themselves being the first to provide first aid, the attitudes of the victims and people involved at the time of the accident are still poorly reported in the literature[17,23,26].

In a survey of 10 Community Health Agents (CHAs), seven of them had already witnessed a situation in which first aid was necessary, such as hyperthermia, firearm injury, hemorrhage, motorcycle accident and convulsion, but they had never received specific training[6].

In another study carried out with candidates for the National Driver's License (CNH), 53% of those interviewed said they had already experienced situations with unconscious victims, more than 34% had witnessed convulsions and more than 32% car accidents. In another population-based study, 72.5% of the subjects said they did not feel prepared to provide first aid[7,27].

In a survey of 188 parents attending a children's hospital who were asked about the care they would give their children in the event of a burn accident, only 10% of all respondents reported appropriate first aid actions. half of them revealed that they had never received specific information or attended a course with this focus[28,29].

This is worrying data, given that lay people often find themselves unable to perform basic first aid measures, and some even report not knowing the telephone number of the urgent and emergency services[27, 29].

In a survey of driver's license applicants, 10% of those interviewed said that the emergency service was Rescue (firefighters) - 193 instead of 192, which would be the Mobile Emergency Assistance Service (SAMU).In another study of high school students, they realized the need to call the emergency service in the event of accidents, but reported difficulty in associating the telephone number with the service, confusing it with the police number[11,27].

Calling the police or fire department would not be at all inappropriate in an emergency situation, since they have specific training to give instructions over the phone, or indicate the appropriate phone number, but in the case of a situation that requires advanced life support, calling the wrong service would be a waste of time with serious consequences that could be avoided[27].

The unpreparedness of the population, both to act immediately when an accident occurs and to request specialized care, is mentioned by the majority of authors. In addition, there are also frequent reports of inappropriate attitudes such as inadequate mobilization manoeuvres, putting the victim at risk. 70% of the participants in one study reported a lack of knowledge when asked to describe block mobilization[6,26,29].

Data from the literature shows that popular approaches in emergency situations and when dealing with wounds are commonly used, such as applying toothpaste, cooking oil, tomato paste, yogurt, milk and egg white to burns, which could increase the risk of infection or slow down the healing process[30,31].

Another difficulty highlighted in the literature is the identification of clinical situations and the measures that could be taken, for example, in Cardiopulmonary Arrest (CA).Two studies have shown that when laypeople notice the absence of breathing and heartbeat, they consider the victim to be dead and do not perform cardiopulmonary resuscitation (CPR) or call an ambulance, but instead call the police because of the difficulty in distinguishing potentially reversible CPR from death[6],[17],[(26)].

In other cases, many of those interviewed would only call for help when there was no longer a pulse or breathing. This corroborates the literature which states that there is a break in the first link in the chain of survival, which corresponds to calling for help before applying any maneuvers[6,32].

When there is a sudden loss of consciousness in an adult, the first thing the rescuer should do is call the emergency medical service. However, in one study, only 31% of respondents called the specialized service when they saw such a situation, and 15% did nothing. In a study of secondary school students, most of them were aware of the signs of CPR, but did not know what to do when they identified it[7,11,26].

There are many barriers that prevent a layperson, trained or not, from acting in an emergency situation, such as the presence of other bystanders, fear of infection or of causing harm to the victim, among other reasons. Only a small proportion provide care because of the fear of harming the victim or contracting a disease[7,8,16].

Training in first aid is a measure that increases the willingness of lay people to help, as they feel safer and more prepared. There are those who consider assisting victims of accidents or injuries to be the sole responsibility of health professionals[7,11,16].

However, the majority of participants in one study, 82.5%, rated first aid training as very important, understanding the concept that anyone can or even should provide care, and that they should at least be trained to do so, without being exclusively a health professional[11,20].

The form adopted by health professionals to disseminate information is called health education and consists of a strategy for social responsibility and the individual's contribution to their own health and that of their peers[20].

Throughout the ages, health education has become one of the government's strategies for ensuring the development of disease control and prevention measures. However, despite the fact that health education is ancient, its action is still currently weak in terms of operationalization, given that health services give little or no importance to educational measures and still focus heavily on curative measures[33].

In addition, educational activities are not being prioritized due to the concept or understanding that health professionals have of health education, or because institutions only give importance to the number of priority visits, leaving activities with the community in the background[34].

At the national level, there is no model program for training laypeople in first aid, just a few isolated actions without a specific focus. Even so, there is a need for more encouragement of this practice, making the population an ally in the fight to preserve public health[27].

Basic rescue measures and CPR maneuvers should be taught to the entire population, because shared knowledge is not reduced, but multiplied, and the population can only benefit from it.

4.2. MEANS OF DISSEMINATING INFORMATION

In addition to the scarcity of studies on laypeople's knowledge of first aid, there are even fewer studies focusing on the profile of people considered unfit to provide first aid. This would be useful in order to infer something about a possible pattern of characteristics.

In the few studies that did exist, the differences in education were not very obvious. In one of them, 67% of those considered unskilled had completed elementary school. Among those considered to be low-skilled, 50% had secondary or higher education (60%). These data do not allow significant differences to be identified[27].

Some authors consider that the level of knowledge is influenced by characteristics such as gender, occupation, area of residence and age, which is considered to be inversely proportional to the ability to provide assistance, since the aging process would determine cognitive alterations[6,7,27].

This information is relevant for identifying priority groups for educational work and also for adapting the means of disseminating information, which will vary according to certain characteristics of the subjects. The lack of adaptation of the means of communication and also of the syllabus of courses and training to the target population has been pointed out as a hindrance to retaining knowledge after completion[26,27].

In a study of 420 children and adolescents, 33% said they had already received information about accident prevention or first aid measures, the main sources of which were school, family, books, medical professionals, the internet and especially television[29].

Children and adolescents are currently very connected to and influenced by electronic media, especially the internet, which can be used as a tool to disseminate important information on various aspects, including health education[35].

Modernity and the large number of means of communication have made it possible to increase the volume of health information available to the population, but the quality of this information, especially that provided on the internet, is often inadequate and inaccurate. It is essential that the information is provided by people who could represent or exercise authority on the subject[35,36].

It is believed that the existence of a reliable *website* on First Aid or Basic Life Support (BLS) could help not only to increase the number of people informed about the correct procedures involved in caring for victims, but also to help diversify the methods and resources used to guide and train people[37].

The dissemination of information by electronic means not only facilitates access because it is widely available at any time, but also because it reduces costs.Nursing students point to the high financial cost as the reason for never having taken part in BLS training, followed by the inconvenience of the courses and the lack of knowledge of their existence, among other reasons[38].

As for the reasons that would encourage students to take part in future training courses, the availability of free courses or charging lower fees and improved accessibility to courses stand out[37].

If the lack of access to information about courses and financial difficulties is already evident among health students, what about the general public, who have fewer sources of information and less motivation to invest financially in this area?

A review of the national literature highlights that, despite the existence of training in BLS, greater investment should be made to facilitate access and the dissemination of information to the largest possible percentage of the population. Technological resources such as videos and websites can be used to disseminate theoretical knowledge about BLS with good assimilation, although it is important to complement this with practical activities to acquire the necessary skills[7,26,37].

A major problem with training courses is the retention of knowledge and skills, as the content taught and the maneuvers are not applied frequently and are difficult to recall. Studies show that knowledge retention begins to decline around two weeks after training and deteriorates around three to six months later[6,9,27].

This highlights the importance not only of training, but also of refresher courses, even if they are sporadic. There is also a need to include the most relevant topics in people's daily lives, such as identifying a CPR; caring for the movement of a person with a suspected spinal fracture; caring for intoxications, convulsions, burns and unconscious victims[27].

This information can be disseminated in a variety of environments such as schools, colleges, workplaces and places where the general public circulates, such as fairs and large events, highlighting the importance of tailoring the information to the target audience[6, 9], [26].

It is important to exclude technical terms from courses aimed at the lay population, as well as from general first aid guidelines in places such as drug leaflets. The technical language used often hinders the proper interpretation of information, making it useless and uninteresting to the public[39].

The illiteracy and/or low level of education of certain groups and the poor access to information contribute to a differentiation in the communication patterns of these people, adopting their own dialects and restricting their level of understanding of more sophisticated terms[39].

A study carried out with rural workers in an agricultural region of Rio de Janeiro found that no worker could understand the First Aid instructions on the label of a herbicide due to the high technical content of the information. They were unable to understand terms such as "inhalation" and "ingestion", which are everyday terms for health professionals and are often used unnoticed without the public understanding[40].

Therefore, it is possible to state that training courses, manuals, programs, leaflets and information in general need to undergo changes in their design, according to the audience they are aimed at, and should be more simplified, containing more targeted information and adapted to the target audience[39].

This highlights the importance and need to invest more effort in creating and disseminating new technologies for first aid training, so that they can be widely used for training and disseminating information, both to health professionals and lay people[37].

4.3. LINES OF ACTION FOR HEALTH EDUCATION

Authors point out that changes in the population's attitudes and behavior when faced with emergency situations are possible through health education. However, they don't happen quickly, but are the result of constant educational work, since adequate prior knowledge implies benefits for both the victims and their families and communities[41].

It is essential to raise awareness of the importance of educating laypeople in order to increase survival, since early access to specialized services can be delayed by their inability to assess the emergency, diagnose situations such as trauma or cardiac arrest and call for help[42].

Studies point to a reduction of up to 7.5% in mortality in pre-hospital settings by teaching the general population first aid gestures in emergency situations, especially through the implementation of CPR training programs in the community[1].

According to data from a survey of patients with heart disease, 86% of cardiac arrests occur in the victims' own homes and are attended by family members, around 50% of whom are children or adolescents. They are a group with great potential for practicing and spreading CPR techniques and other first aid measures[1, 43].

Education is a building process that requires time, dedication and continuity, so it needs to start at an early age and therefore the first notions of accident prevention and first aid should be introduced at an early age[16].

According to the European Resuscitation Council, first aid training courses should include: rescuer safety, diagnosis of CPR by means of arresponsiveness and abnormal breathing, CPR and proper mobilization of the victim [(44).]

The success of out-of-hospital CPR depends on early diagnosis of CPR, activation of the emergency services, immediate start of CPR and rapid defibrillation. These procedures represent the links in the chain of survival that has the potential and fundamental participation of the bystander[1].

Activating the emergency service, the first step in the link, as well as allowing for the rapid dispatch of basic or advanced ambulance support, as necessary, can provide guidance for trained first responders or not, facilitating the care of the victim[1].

In addition, the production and socialization of knowledge about first aid can lead to a reduction in the demand considered not pertinent to the SAMU, making it more efficient and optimizing emergency care for those who really need it[16].

Another important action aimed at speeding up and making effective the first emergency care provided by laypeople would be to make Automated External Defibrillators (AEDs) available in places where people are crowded. This equipment is simple to use and is capable of monitoring the cardiac activity of victims, identifying the type of cardiac arrest, determining the need for defibrillation and applying it when necessary [45].

It is a huge advance over CPR and can be used in the out-of-hospital environment by any trained rescuer. However, despite the recognized importance of using the AED in the out-of-hospital environment and the fact that there is specific state legislation, based on national legislation, to make it available in places of movement, this equipment is still not easily accessible to the population[45].

Perhaps facts like this are due to the idea that equipment such as an AED and CPR training are not necessary, as it is imagined that a situation such as CPR will never occur in certain places. However, as these situations are often unpredictable, giving up equipment such as an AED could mean one or more potentially avoidable deaths occurring.

First aid training for laypeople should basically educate the population to recognize an emergency situation and decide on the best course of action to take while waiting for specialized help[20,23,26].

Training programs must eliminate the factors that inhibit the willingness to apply BLS maneuvers, and increase the spectator's willingness to act and the quality of this action, with the safety and skill to do so[6,23].

The standardization of care to be followed is the responsibility of health professionals, institutions and the population itself, when exercising their citizenship. It is also important to continue training in the basics of first aid, starting in places such as schools, thus promoting health education from the earliest stages. Providing information and training in first aid means encouraging the formation of individuals who are more autonomous, supportive and prepared to contribute to society [11,20].

5. FINAL CONSIDERATIONS

In this literature review, in line with the hypothesis developed, few studies were found on laypeople's knowledge of first aid. The selected studies showed that the majority of the groups studied had incomplete or inadequate knowledge, which could compromise first aid and cause harm to the victims being assisted.

The findings were worrying given that many emergency situations are witnessed and assisted by lay people, such as family members and passers-by who, if properly trained, could act as allies in preserving the lives and physical integrity of other people, representing a social commitment.

We highlight the strategies for health education, such as adapting the means of disseminating information, the content and the terms according to the target audience, in order to make the most of and understand the information, as well as implementing educational actions from an early age, using the school as a suitable place for this.

It would be interesting to carry out other studies on the knowledge of laypeople involving other audiences, or perhaps even a population-based study with this focus so that we can better elucidate the factors that promote and hinder learning first aid measures.

A situational diagnosis is the first step towards formulating and implementing effective health education strategies for the lay public. So that, as well as feeling empowered to act in emergency situations, they become multipliers of knowledge.

REFERENCES

1. AMERICAN HEART ASSOCIATION. International Liaison Committee on Resuscitation. Guidelines 2000 for Cardiopulmonary Resuscitation and Emergency Cardiovascular Care. Part 4: the automated external defibrillator: key link in the chain of survival. Circulation, Stanford, v. 102, n. 8 (suppl.), p. 160-176, 2000.

2. MAIA, E.R et al. Knowledge of Pre-Hospital Care and Basic Life Support by New Medical Students. Revista Brasileira de Educagao M6dica, 38 (1): 59-64; Ceara, 2014.

3. BRAZIL, Ministry of Health. First Aid Manual. Oswaldo Cruz Foundation. FIOCRUZ. Rio de Janeiro, 2003.

4. MARQUES, M.D;JUNIOR, L.C.L;BOMFIM, E.O et al. The teaching of first aid from the perspective of a problem-oriented curriculum. J. res.: fundam. care. Online, Oct./Dec. 6(4):1485-1495, 2014.

5. BASTOS, J.J.C. Crime of omission of aid: interpretative divergences and critical observations. Revista Brasileira de Ciencias Criminais, (34): 45-62, Apr./Jun. Sao Paulo: RT, 2001.

6. VENTORINI, J.A.L;BADKE, M.R;COGO, S.B; COSENTINO, S.F; Santos, V.O. Conhecimentos e conduta dos Agentes Comunitarios de Saude frente aos primeiros socorros. Rev Enferm UFSM, May/Aug;2(2):353-364, 2012.

7. PERGOLA, A.M;ARAUJO, I.E.M. O leigo e o suporte basico de vida. Rev Esc Enferm USP, 43(2): 335-42, 2009.

8. BERG, R.A; HEMPHILL, R; ABELLA, B.S;AUFDERHEIDE, T.P;CAVE, D.M;HAZINSKI, M.F; LERNER, E.B; REA, T.D; SAYRE, M.R; SWOR, R.A. Part 5: Adult Basic Life Support 2010 American Heart Association Guidelines for

Cardiopulmonary Resuscitation and Emergency Cardiovascular Care. Circulation. 2010.

9. BOAVENTURA,A.P;COUTINHO, R.M.C. Suporte basico de vida: conhecimento dos profissionais de ambulatorios de saude ocupacional. Proceedings of the 10th Latin American Scientific Initiation Meeting and 6th Latin American Postgraduate Meeting; 2006 Oct 19-20; Sao Josd dos Campos. Sao Paulo; p. 2748-51, 2006.

10. TIMERMAN, S;MORAIS, D.A; CARVALHO, D.V;GONZALEZ,M.M.C. Cardiorespiratory arrest in the prehospital environment: occurrences attended by the mobile emergency care service of Belo Horizonte. Rev Bras Clin Med. Belo Horizonte, 7:211-8, 2009.

11. SILVA, P.O; OLIVEIRA, T.G.S; MARTA, C.B;FRANCISCO, M.T.R; MARTINS, E.R.C; SAMPAIO, C.E,P. High school students and their knowledge of basic life support. Rev. enferm. UERJ, Rio de Janeiro; 20(esp.1):621-4, dec 2012.

12. COCCO, M.; LOPES M.J.M. Violence among young people: social

dynamics and situations of vulnerability. Rev. Gaucha Enferm., v.31, n.1, p.151-9, 2010.

13. BRAZIL. Health Portal. Types and Nature of Violence. Brasilia (DF). *[website*
Available at: http://www.portal.saude.gov.brAcesso *on May 25, 2015.*

14. VIALLE, E.N; VIALLE, L.R; TORRES, L.F.B; SAKAMOTO, K.S . Histological evaluation of the effect of methylprednisolone on experimental spinal cord injury in rats. Revista Brasileira de Ortopedia, Varosoft, April, 2007.

15. GONZAGA, R.A.T; RIMOLI, C.F; PIRES, E.A; ZOGHEIB, F,S; FUJINO, M.V.T; CUNHA, M.B. Avaliagao da mortalidade por causas externas. Rev. Col. Bras. Cir. vol.39 no.4 Rio de Janeiro July/Aug. 2012.

16. VERONESE, A.M; OLIVEIRA, D.L.L.C; ROSA, I.M; NAST, K. First aid workshops: experience report. Rev Gaucha Enferm., Porto Alegre (RS); 31(1):179-82, Mar 2010.

17. ALVES, T.S; COGO, A.L. Seeking evidence for training in basic life support - a systematic literature review. Online Braz.j. nurs. (Online); 5(2), 2006.

18. BERNARDES, E.L; MACIEL, F.A; DEL VECCHIO, F.B. First aid at school: level of knowledge of teachers in the city of Monte Mor.Movimento e Percepgao, Espirito Santo do Pinhal, v. 8, n. 11, 2007.

19. HAFEN, Q; KARREN, J.K; FRANDSEN, J.K. First aid for students.

Barueri: Malone, 2002.

20. FIORUC, B.E; MOLINA, A.C; JUNIOR, W.V;LIMA, S.A.M. Educação em saúde: abordando primeiros socorros em escolas públicas no interior de Sao Paulo. Rev. Eletr. Enf. 10(3): 695-702,2008.

21. SIQUEIRA, G.S; SOARES, L.A; SANTOS, R.A. Atuação do professor de educagao fisica diante de situações de primeiros socorros. EFDeportes.com, Digital Magazine. Buenos Aires, N. 154, March 2011.

22. GOEL, S; SINGH, N; LAL, V; SINGH, A. Knowledge, attitude and practices of students about first aid epilepsy seizures management in a Northern Indian City. Ann Indian Acad Neurol;16:538-43, 2013.

23. VECCHIO, F.B.D; VECCHIO, A.H.M.D; BLANCO, B.F.V; GONCALVES, A. Training in first aid: an intervention study in the school environment. Cadernos de Formagao RBCE, p. 56-70, mar. 2010.

24. SAMPAIO, R.F; MANCINI, M.C. Systematic Review Studies: A guide for the careful synthesis of scientific evidence. Rev. bras. fisioter., Sao Carlos, v. 11, n. 1, p. 83-89, jan./feb. 2007.

25. MINAYO, M.C.S. O desafio do conhecimento - pesquisa qualitativa em saude , 11.ed. Sao Paulo: Hucitec, 2008.

26. PERGOLA, A.M; ARAUJO, I.E.M. O leigo em situagoes de emergencia. Rev Esc Enf USP;42(4)769-76, 2008.

27. MARCONATO, A.M.P. First aid course for candidates for the National Driver's License. Doctoral thesis presented to the Postgraduate Program in Nursing, Faculty of Nursing, State University of Campinas. Campinas-SP, 2003.

28. GRAHAM, H.E, BACHE, S.E; MUTHA,Y.Y.A. P; BAKER, J; RALSTON, D.R. Are parents in the UK equipped to provide adequate burns first aid? Burns. 38(3):438-43, 2012.

29. GONCALVES, A.C.G; ECHEVARRIA-GUANILO, M.E; GONCALVES, N; ROSSI, L.A; FARINA JUNIOR, J.A. Characterization of patients treated in a burn service and attitudes at the time of the accident. Rev. Eletr. Enf. 14(4):866-72, oct/dec. 2012.

30. HODGINS, P; POTOKAR, T; PRICE, P. Comparing rich and poor: Burn prevention in Wales, Pakistan, India, Botswana and Zambia. Burns. 37:1354-59, 2011.

31. HARVEY, L.A; BARR, M.L; POULOS, R.G; FINCH, C.F; SHERKER, S; HARVEY, J.G. A population-based survey of knowledge of first aid for burns in New South Wales. Med J Aust.195(8):465-8, 2011.

32. AMERICAN HEART ASSOCIATION. Highlights from the 2010 American Heart Association guidelines for CPR and ACE. Mary Fran Hazinski, editor. 2010. Available at: ftp://ftp.medicina.ufmg.br/ped/arquivos/Novas guidelines.pdf

33. SABOIA, V.M. A Enfermeira e a pratica educativa em saude: a arte de talhar pedras. Rev Nurs.83(8):173-7, 2005.

34. MELO, G; SANTOS, R.M; TREZZA, M.C.S.F. Entendimento e pratica de agoes educativas de profissionais do Programa Saude da Familia de Sao Sebastiao-AL: detectando dificuldades. Rev Bras Enferm.58(3):290-

5, 2005.

35. OLIVEIRA, M.C.A.M; PAULO, M.M. Influencia da media no processo de desenvolvimento do adolescente. Revista cientifica eletonica de psicologia. Year VI, Number 10, 2008.

36. HSIAO, M; TSAI, B; UK, P; JO, H; GOMEZ, M; GOLLOGLY, J.G et al. "What do kids know": A survey of 420 Grade 5 students in Cambodia on their knowledge of burn prevention and first-aid treatment. Burns. 33(3):347-51, 2007.

37. MORI, S; WHITAKER, I.Y; MARIN, H.F. Evaluation of the First Aid educational *website*. Rev Esc Enferm USP. 47(4):950-7, 2013.

38. LIBERMAN, M; GOLBERG, N; MEULDER, D; SAMPALIS, J. Teaching cardiopulmonary resuscitation to CEGEP students in Quebec: a pilot project. Resuscitation. 47(3)249-57, 2000.

39. TOMAZIN, C.C; ZAMBRONE, F.A.D. Level of understanding of first-aid information on agrochemical leaflets and labels by tomato farmers in Sumard, SP. Revista Brasilcira de Toxicologia 21, n.1 (20 - 24), 2008.

40. MOREIRA, J.C; JACOB, S; PERES, F; LIMA, J.S; MEYE, R.A; OLIVEIRA-SILVA, J.J et al. Integrated evaluation of the impact of pesticide use on human health in an agricultural community in Nova Friburgo, RJ. Ciencia & Saude Coletiva 2002; 7: 299-31.

41. SHAN, M.U; GAKRISHNAN, R.R; NARAYANAN, V; THIRUMA,

L.A; IKOLUNDU, S; UBRAMANI, A.N.P. Epidemiology of burns in a teaching hospital in south India. Indian J Plast Surg. 41(1):34-37, 2008.

42. FERREIRA, D.F;TIMERMAN, A;STAPLETON, E;TIMERMAN, S; RAMIRES,J.A.F. Practical application of teaching in medical emergencies. Rev Soc Cardiol Estado de Sao Paulo.11(2):505-11, 2011.

43. FEITOSA-FILHO, G.S; FEITOSA, G.F; GUIMARAES, H.P; LOPES, R.D;
MORAES- JUNIOR, R; SOUTO, F.A; VASQUES, R; TIMERMAN, S. Update on cardiopulmonary resuscitation: what has changed with the new guidelines! [internet journal] 2006 [cited 2012 Sep 13]; 18(2):177-85. Available at:
http://www.scielosp.org/pdf/rbti/v18n2/a11v18n2.pdf.

44. SOAR, J; MONSIEURS, K.G;BALANCE, J.H.W; BARELLI, A; BIARENT, D; GREIF, R.et al. EuropeanResuscitation Council Guidelines for Resuscitation 2010 - Section 9. Principles of education in resuscitation. Resuscitation. 81(10):1434-44, 2010.

45. Sao Paulo. State Law No. 12736, of October 2007. Regulates the availability of defibrillators in places where people gather. [Accessed June 2, 2013]. Available at:http://www.cremesp.org.br/?siteAcao=legislagao&id=415

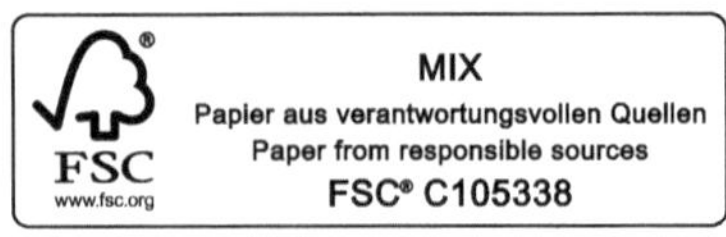

Printed by Books on Demand GmbH, Norderstedt / Germany